The Not-so-Scary
Breast
c a n c e r
Book

Two Sisters' Guide from Discovery to Recovery

Carolyn Ingram, Ed.D.
Leslie Ingram Gebhart, M.A.

Illustrated by Mary Clark

Impact ◆ Publis
ATASCADERO, CALIFO.

D0006624

ATTENTION ORGANIZATIONS AND CORPORATIONS:
This book is available at quantity discounts on bulk purchases for educational, business, or sales promotional use. For further information, please contact Impact Publishers, P.O. Box 6016, Atascadero, California 93423-6016. Phone: 1-800-246-7228. e-mail: sales@impactpublishers.com

Photograph of Carolyn Ingram by Stuart Schwartz.
Photograph of Leslie Ingram Gebhart and Mary Clark by Joan Lauren.

Library of Congress Cataloging-in-Publication Data

Ingram, Carolyn
   The not-so-scary breast cancer book : two sisters' guide from discovery to recovery / Carolyn Ingram, Leslie Gebhart : illustrated by Mary Clark.
         p.   cm.
   Includes bibliographical references and index.
   ISBN: 1-886230-29-3 (alk. paper)
      1. Breast--Cancer Popular works.   I. Gebhart, Leslie. II. Title.
RC280.B81534   1999
616.99'449--dc21   99-37875
                                                                         CIP

Impact Publishers and colophon are registered trademarks of Impact Publishers, Inc.
Cover design by Sharon Schnare, San Luis Obispo, California
Printed in the United States of America on acid-free paper
Published by *Impact ✍ Publishers*®
POST OFFICE BOX 6016
ATASCADERO, CALIFORNIA 93423-6016
www.impactpublishers.com

Thanks to our children teachers,
Leslie Ann,
Craig, Gare,
Karin, and Courtney.

Hugs and appreciation
to
Bob and David.

Contents

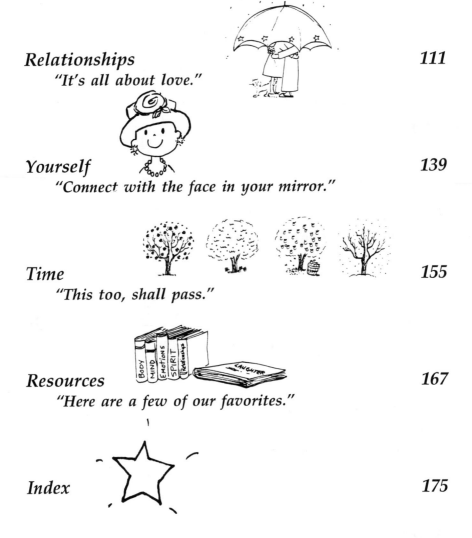

*A sense of well-being embodies
balance — a connecting and intertwining
of the body, emotions, mind,
spirit and relationships in ways
that create equipoise. We'll
emphasize this interrelatedness
as we offer hints for coping with
a cancer diagnosis.*

PREFACE

The intention of this book is to provide comfort and inspiration both to those who have received a cancer diagnosis and the people in their lives. Our experience is with breast cancer.

Chaos and confusion came first for us. As time went by, we began talking about what helped and what didn't help. In some cases, what Carolyn needed was very different from what Leslie needed. The differences as much as the similarities in our experience guided us to what we believe to be universal. We want to help you find what you need and avoid some of the pitfalls during this difficult time.

In general, fear and terror subside as time passes after the diagnosis and treatment. There are times the reality of coping with cancer does interrupt—it has become a fact of life. For now, that's how it is. You aren't cancer. You are much much more—you are many faceted. Think about whatever helps you to feel love. Celebrate your specialness, your uniqueness. We hope this book will add to the light you already shine.

Much of what is to follow is general information we cherish. The "we" are sisters, Carolyn and Leslie.

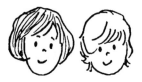

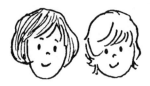

We both have been physically fit and health conscious with no family history of breast cancer. When our perspectives are the same, we use this type style. Often we agree. When our perspectives are different, or when we are sharing our individual experience, we changed type styles to indicate which voice you are reading—that of

Carolyn, who had a lumpectomy, chemotherapy, and radiation. Carolyn found her own lump.

Leslie, who had bilateral mastectomy. Mammogram found Leslie's.

Our friend and illustrator, Mary, interprets our words with heartfelt drawings.

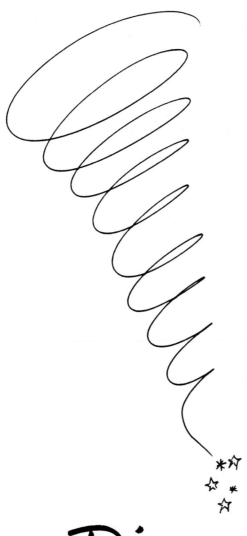

Discovery

" ... but cancer doesn't run in my family... "

DISCOVERY

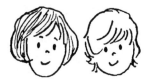

We both had an irrational but understandable wish: not to literally turn back the clock, but to retrieve the innocence, the confidence and the ease of mind of looking at life through the eyes of someone who did not have cancer.

For me it would have been the moment before I found the lump. That moment was followed by a sense of unreality, of weakness in the knees, of preoccupation that kept me from being fully present to myself and my daughter. It blocked my field of vision as surely as if it were a ball in front of my eyes around which I tried to peek at the world.

For me it was hearing the diagnosis from the surgeon. I froze with dark fear, oppressive and panicky blackness that threatened to block my view of the sunshine, of life continuing.

This was the bleakest time for us. It may be a time when you can not find your own strength. Accept that for now, and don't add another worry.

At the time of diagnosis, I lived with my school-aged daughter and husband and had a part-time private psychology practice so I could be an "at home" mom while my husband worked. The shock of diagnosis derailed me completely. My urgency was to have the surgery and start treatment immediately. Because of node involvement, I needed chemotherapy. I chose lumpectomy and radiation instead of mastectomy. The process took approximately six months. My doctor recommended a therapist who had breast cancer nearly ten years earlier. She said, "Some day you will look back at this as the year you had cancer." Hearing that was my first ray of hope that there would be a time I wouldn't be in shock. My sister, Leslie, became an important part of my support team. I am the younger sister.

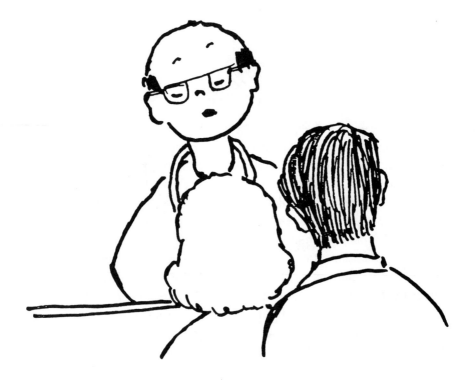

 My husband and I heard the cancer diagnosis from the surgeon the day after the biopsy.

At the time of diagnosis, I was in a comfortable "empty nest" routine with my husband of more than thirty years. I had a part time career as a writer/publisher and enjoyed frequent visits with our two adult children who live in another city. From reading my sister's introduction, I identify most readily with the words, "urgency" and "immediately." I read the material my doctor recommended, scurried around my medical community, heard five of five concurring opinions and chose mastectomy. I am the "first born," though the second to receive a cancer diagnosis. Approximately one year after Carolyn completed her treatment, she became the support person for me — role changing of a unique kind.

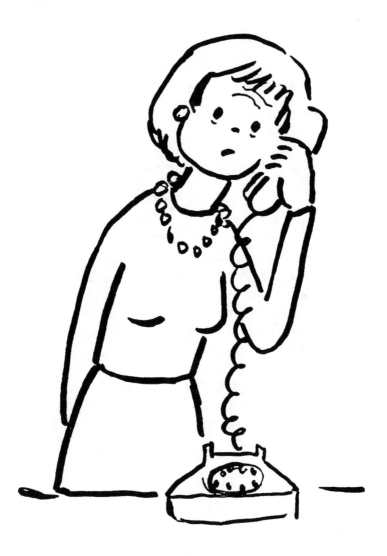

 I heard, ". . . the diagnosis is breast cancer . . ." over the telephone.

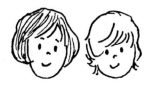

No matter what treatment you select, you may
second guess your decision. So did we.

Cancer is a fact - part of
what now gets your attention -
but you are not cancer.
Cancer does not extinguish
your light.

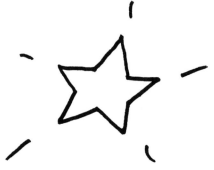

General Hints for Coping At Diagnosis Time

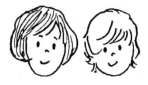

A diagnosis forces us to take action.

Accept that you will be spending more time with medical matters and that may have an emotional impact.

Make your needs known, first to yourself, then to others. If this is hard for you, especially when you are so vulnerable, know that that's normal. This is the time to ask those you trust to help you know what you need and help you to ask for it.

Choose/do what it takes to find out how you feel more nurtured and empowered and less scared.

Practice being as kind to yourself as you would be to a dear friend.

Some patients want to read and to know everything; some want to rely on their doctor's knowledge and expertise. Both are healthy ways to cope. As you read this, notice which feels right to you. (We've included a short list of our favorite readings on the subject in the "Resources" section at the end of the book.)

Working with medical personnel and sensing yourself as part of the team can become part of your personal healing journey.

Feel your power when it is time to make a decision. It is your body, your experience, your life, your choice.

Fear, Anxiety, Numbness

Until we receive the diagnosis none of us knows what our reaction will be. Panic, worry, fearfulness, numbness, sadness are just a few "normal" responses we experience. Wanting to sleep a lot or not being able to sleep at all are common during the time right after diagnosis and before treatment. Accept that there is a range of responses and many ways to find help.

If you are reading this after your decisions have been made, remember it's "normal" to second guess yourself. If you don't have chemotherapy, you begin to wonder if you should have had it. If you chose a lumpectomy over mastectomy, you may feel the need to keep checking breast tissue. If you do or if you do not take certain drugs, you may think you shouldn't or should. If you chose mastectomy, you re-wonder if it should have been a bilateral. If you had bilateral, you wonder if all the breast tissue is really gone. All this is normal process. You can find support for any choice. Hearing contradictory opinions is common and can be confusing or seem overwhelming. Select carefully those with whom you discuss your situation.

You may need things
you haven't needed before.

Making Choices

Ambiguity and worry and anxiety about the choices that need to be made are natural. Don't worry about worrying. Indecisiveness is natural too. If you feel stuck while needing to make a decision, ask for help.

Even when your choices seem limited, involve fear, disease and make you feel fragile or vulnerable, taking action can be freeing. There are big decisions such as lumpectomy? mastectomy? drug therapy? chemo? radiation? Once those are made, there are smaller decisions such as time and day for treatment and what kind of support you want.

Face difficult decisions, gather facts, then do that which seems right. Difficult choices are less burdensome once made.

Making choices
was a relief for me.

Making choices
energized me.

If you are anxious, find out what helps you to manage worry:

1. scheduling a doctor's appointment
2. meditating*
3. writing in a journal
4. going to group*
5. going to a therapist
6. finding a guide for visualization*
7. talking to a friend
8. changing the rhythm of your breath
9. praying

If you take one path — and you don't like what you find there — or, you hear new information that causes you to question your choice, you can take a different path.

I found my therapist through an acquaintance who had breast cancer. Ask friends or your doctor for recommendations of people who specialize in breast cancer. This will probably lead you to someone you too will like.

---

* Throughout this book, we have used this symbol to call attention to material that can be found in the Resources section of the book.

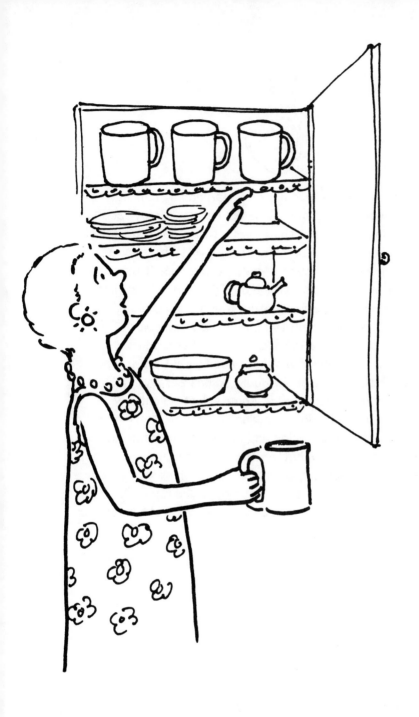

Reaching for things in the kitchen like the paper towels or cups in the cupboard is one way to stretch.

Wigs

The hardest part of all this was hearing I had breast cancer. The second hardest was hearing that I needed chemotherapy because of lymph node involvement. The third hardest was learning that the kind of chemo I needed would also cause my hair to fall out. A friend accompanied me to several wig shops. Because it was near Halloween, other shoppers were trying on "fright" wigs and there was lots of laughing. I left crying. Later I found a specialist. She brought scarfs, hats and a variety of wig styles and colors. Even though I had not looked good in hats, she found several that looked great. As with people who choose not to wear prostheses, some people wear their baldness proudly, some wear a wig all the time to look as "normal" as possible, some select an entirely different "look," and others do a combination of hat, scarf, bald, wig varying it to suit the situation and mood. Many beauty salons have wig services to help. No matter what you think, if I can wear a hat, anyone can. If you can't find hats that you think look good, ask someone to help you. There is a hat that's the right shape for you even if you don't think so now. At night I wore a cotton hat for warmth and recommend it.

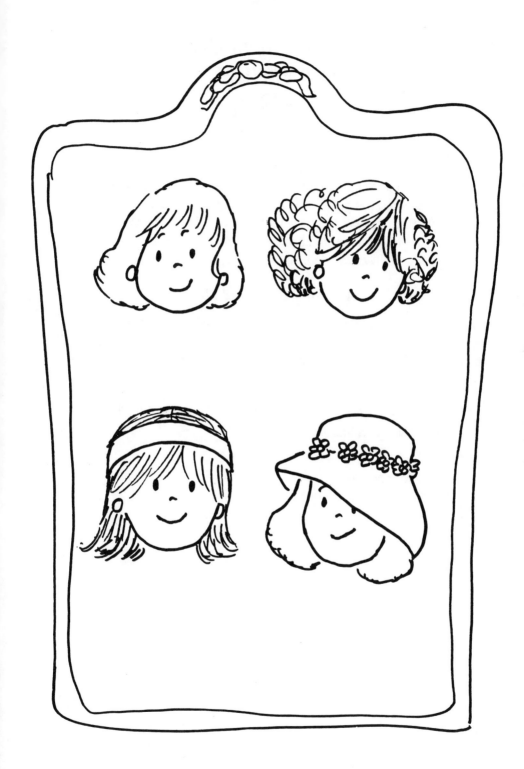

Complementary Treatment Considerations

Acupuncture helped me to get through surgery, chemotherapy and radiation. I trust that acupuncture does balance the body and keep energy moving. I also felt very safe and nurtured with my acupuncturist. I believe I got back to "normal" faster because of acupuncture and the herbs I took. I consulted with my doctors about the herbs I was taking.

Avoiding Colds and Flu

When in chemotherapy you are more susceptible to infections. It is very important to avoid colds and flu. Taking extra caution at this time is important. I did things that were different for me and stayed healthy:

- I slept in a different room when my husband had a cold.
- I washed my hands often.
- I didn't share lip gloss or water bottles.
- I hugged more than kissed that winter and avoided the seasonal bugs my family caught.
- I got a flu shot.

Reconstruction

Before my bilateral surgery, the surgeon wanted to discuss implants. I didn't. I still don't. They're not for me. I chose not to start the implant process at the time of my surgery, agreeing instead to have an appointment one year from the date of surgery to revisit the issue with the surgeon. I have not changed my mind and, frankly, if and when I do want to wear boobs, I enjoy going to the drawer of options to decide which size shoulder pad or breast prosthesis will be most flattering for the particular outfit I'm selecting. For the small-breasted look, shoulder pads work great — especially the kind with the little velcro strips which stay put inside a t-shirt or sports bra. For a larger-breasted look, many options are available, including custom designed and a variety of "off the shelf" styles. To learn more, visit the prostheses department of a health supply store. I found a compassionate and competent fitter who was helpful both in introducing me to the options available and for easing me into the reality of my new chest area.

To reconstruct or not has been a major topic among those in my support group who had mastectomies. The range includes those who planned reconstruction no matter what and those who knew that they were not going to do it no matter what. The majority were in between and decided to wait a year before the final decision. Of these, after several years, no one has chosen reconstruction.

Scar Pain

For many people, healing after surgery is routine and relatively pain free. Mine wasn't. The pain in my scar area was significant and I tolerated it way too long before asking for help, because I didn't know what "normal" healing was. I developed keloids which usually do not occur after an incision. If they do occur, there is help. Ask — insist — if your scars hurt, let your care-givers know so you can get help. I have alternated between regular scar attention and resisting the advice to massage the area with healing creams.

Breast Self Exam

Even though I found the lump during a regular monthly check, after treatment, I developed an irrational fear of continuing these breast checks. I talked with my oncologist who smiled and said, "That's understandable. Do it anyway."

Some things are hard to do.

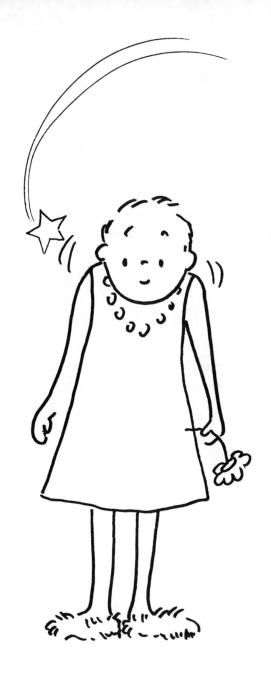

After checking with your Doctor,
wiggle and rotate your shoulders.

Mixed Feelings

When my hair fell out was a low point. It was impossible to pretend everything was okay. On the other hand, it made me know that the chemo was working to kill any cancer cells that might have been left. It is hard, but true, that I am grateful for the toxic chemicals.

Rolling over on soft sheets without soft breasts was a shock. I felt very sad because I missed my boobs. Yet, after the surgery to remove the part that had cancer, I am grateful to have life and health.

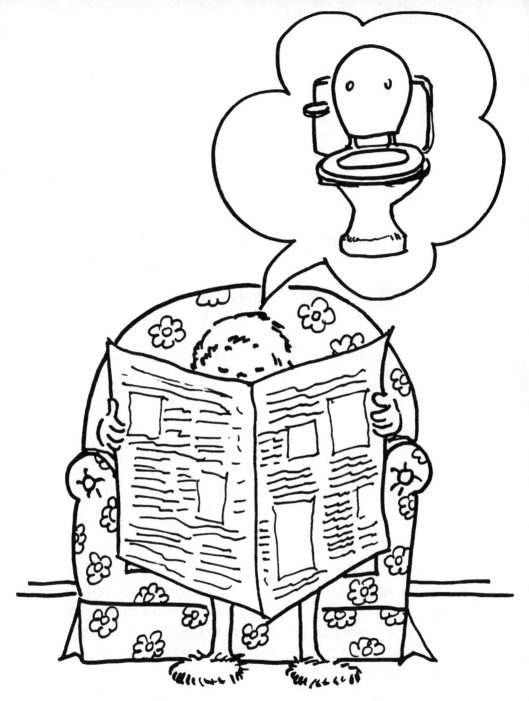

Constipation can result from chemotherapy and is considered "normal" after anesthesia. Ask your doctor what to do.

Deepen your breathing while relaxing your neck and shoulders.

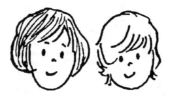

You will notice breathing is mentioned often. We are still learning to remember to breathe consciously. It helps us stay in the present moment. Breathing with intention also brings to our awareness the interconnection of body, mind, spirit, and relationships.

Emotions

" ... it's a rollercoaster.' ... "

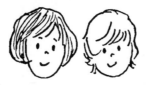

Practice acknowledging emotions as they occur. "If you worry a lot, try instead to feel your other feelings."*

For most, fear comes with a cancer diagnosis — fear of pain, death, recurrence, treatment, surgery, chemo, anesthesia, radiation as well as subtler fears. We found our fears hard to discuss at first — especially the fear of death. Eventually, discussion became an experience of healing for us. One of the goals is to manage fear so it doesn't take over. It is important to learn to discern the kind of fear that tells you something is wrong, and the kind of fear that needs to be shelved. If your fear tells you something is wrong, consult your doctor (even if you're afraid to do so).

I needed to talk with empathetic and reassuring people when I was afraid. It helped me to be carried emotionally by the love, hope and faith of loved ones. Other things that helped were:

- finding the right support group
- finding a therapist who had had breast cancer
- going to a guided visualization specialist where I learned to construct a box that could contain my fear

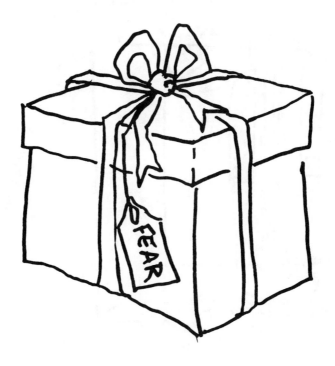

As time passed, I was able to tie closed the fear box, a symbol to contain my fear.

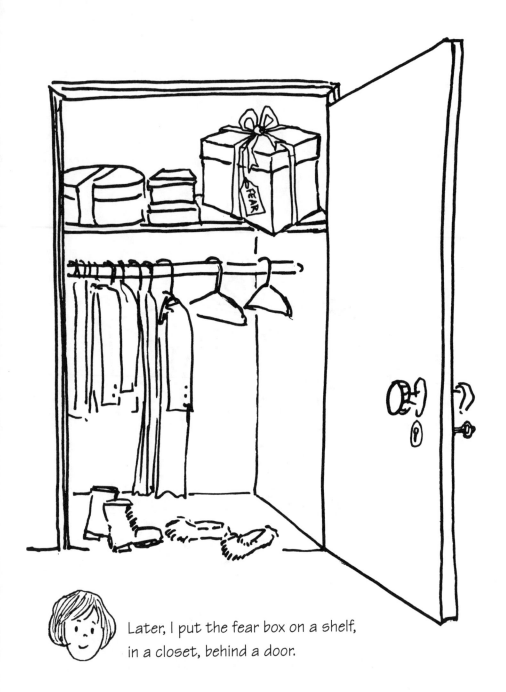

Later, I put the fear box on a shelf, in a closet, behind a door.

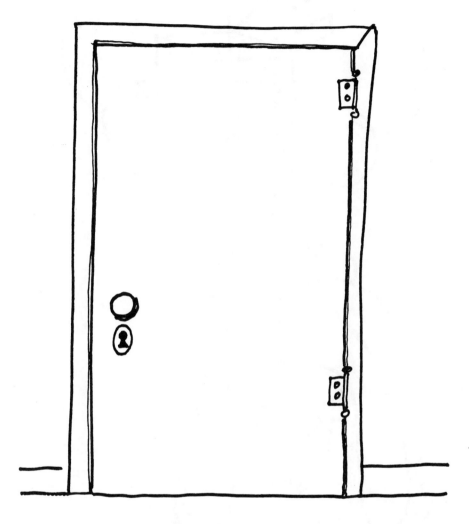

Finally, the fear box was put on a shelf, in a closet, behind a door that was closed and locked with a key symbolizing that though still there, fear was no longer "in my face," dominating life.

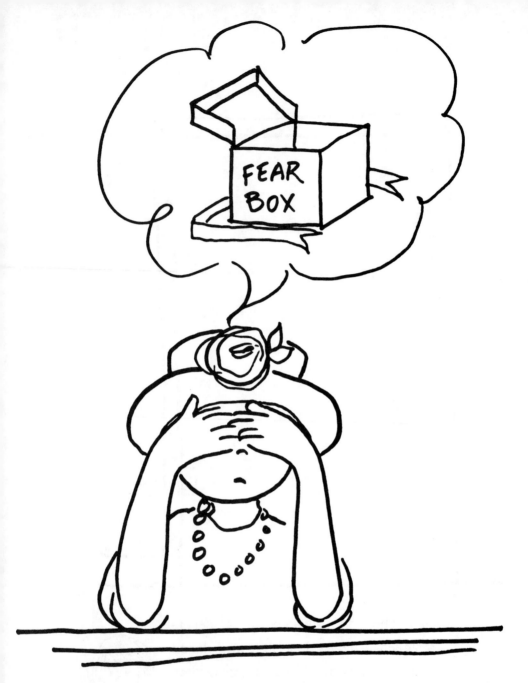

Fear still comes out of the box and seeps under the locked door.